D0723171

A Guide To The BACH FLOWER REMEDIES

by
JULIAN BARNARD

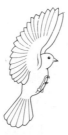

THE C.W. DANIEL COMPANY LTD.
1 Church Path, Saffron Walden
Essex, England.

First published in Great Britain in 1979
© Julian Barnard 1979
All rights reserved
Reprinted 1981, 1983, 1984 and 1985
New edition 1986

The photograph of Gorse on the cover:
by the author.

Printed in Great Britain by
Hillman Printers, Frome, Somerset.

Contents

Introduction	5
The Flower Remedies	8
The Healing Power of Nature	12
How the Remedies Work	14
When we take a Remedy	20
Diagnosis and Prescribing	25
The Twelve Healers and Other Remedies	26
Recognising the Remedy	35
Combination Remedies	41
Dowsing	43
Learning to Diagnose	45
Making the Medicine	49
Bibliography	51

In the name of the One God may the gift of healing be given to all who seek to help those in need.

INTRODUCTION

What are the Bach Remedies? They are a simple and natural method of healing through the use of certain wild flowers. The remedies, which treat the personality disorders of the patient rather than the individual physical condition, were discovered in the 1930s by Dr Edward Bach. After many years of practice in conventional medicine as well as homoeopathy Edward Bach was led to the realisation that what characterised the physical disorders of different people was not so much the many categories of disease but the psychological conditions that generate them. Over a period of years he was enabled to recognise these psychological conditions and find in each case an appropriate remedy. The remedies were found in the flowers of the field and the trees of the countryside — in nature's God-given healing power.

Man has always made use of medicinal herbs. Until recent years all pharmaceutical preparations relied upon the use of natural substances. The Bach Remedies, however, do not use the physical material of the plant but rather the essential energy that is found within the flower. This healing energy is extracted in a particular way and stored in a preserving liquid. This subtle substance is used to treat the cause of illness at the subtle level. By this it is meant that while most medicine treats the physical complaint with a physical material the Bach Remedies treat the unseen or psychological cause with an unseen energy.

In the field of what is popularly called 'alternative medicine' there are forms of healing that are more or less in sympathy with Dr Bach's discoveries. And it is well to stress that no one form of healing has the privilege of being the best or the most effective; everything is appropriate in its own way. It is apparent, however, that Bach's discoveries represent a revolutionary approach to medicine. It may be summed up in his dictum: "treat the patient, not the disease". For no matter what the patient is suffering from in the physical body — it might be asthma or athlete's foot — the prime cause of that condition can be eradicated if we can ascertain and counteract the imbalance that is in the psyche of the patient.

An example will demonstrate how this relationship works in practice. Suppose that two people, in no way related, both receive a deep shock. One of them is involved in a car crash perhaps. She is badly shaken but not physically injured. In the weeks that follow she suffers from constant headaches and nausea. The second fictitious character is a banker who suffers a sudden and severe reversal of his financial fortunes. He has a stroke on hearing the news which results in the partial paralysis of his right arm. The treatments that might be given for these two physical conditions would normally vary. But if we treat the patients' psychological state it would be apparent that they were both suffering from shock though its manifestation in the body was different. Following Dr Bach's methods we would begin by prescribing *Star of Bethlehem* the remedy for all kinds of sudden distress, upsets and accidents. When the shock is neutralised the physical effect will dissolve and disappear.

6

In a similar way a person who suffers from jealousy or fear, from self-pity or resentment may manifest that psychological state in a variety of ways physically. Jealousy may be the root cause of a cancer or pleurisy, self-pity may bring a person out in spots, cause migraine or back-ache. The physical complaint is not important: it is the psychological state that is to be treated.

It might be argued that this is a simplistic view of illness. To quote Dr Bach "it is its simplicity, combined with its all-healing effects, that is so wonderful". In a later section we can try to look at how the remedies work but at this point the necessary question is: "Do they work?" And the answer is quite clearly "Yes". Inevitably there are some diseases which lie beyond the scope of this form of medicine and some conditions which are more suited to other methods of treatment but as we shall see the Bach Remedies can be usefully applied in almost all circumstances.

THE FLOWER REMEDIES

Although there are thousands of variations in physical illness the psychological causes are relatively few. The Bach Remedies recognise 38 conditions each specifically aligned to one of the states that generate 'dis-ease' within the psyche (a description of these 38 remedies is found on p. 26ff.). They are classified under seven headings:

For Fear

For Uncertainty

For Insufficient Interest in Present Circumstances

For Loneliness

For Those Over-sensitive to Influences and Ideas

For Despondency and Despair

For Overcare for the Welfare of Others

Each category covers a range of mental and emotional states. Those concerned with fear, for instance, range from sheer terror (*Rock Rose*), to specific fears like a fear of heights or a fear of animals (*Mimulus*), to anxiety for the anticipated misfortunes of others (*Red Chestnut*). The remedies for despondency and despair range from a feeling of inadequacy (*Larch*) to a remedy that helps in that time of anguish that is sometimes called 'the dark night of the soul' (*Sweet Chestnut*).

Bach found the remedies by searching the countryside for those plants which he instinctively knew were suitable to help specific psychological states. The classification of these states was arrived at by careful observation of human nature and more especially by observation of the way that different people react when suffering from an illness or when under stress. They are of two kinds: there are the Type Remedies which relate to a characteristic type of personality and the Helping Remedies which deal with the transient mood of the psyche. The latter describe conditions which are not necessarily essential to a person's character but which have developed a strong hold upon them. Thus the remedy *Gorse* which is for hopelessness and despair cannot be said to be a characteristic type though it may be the all-pervading condition of the psyche at a particular time. Similarly *Wild Rose*, the remedy for apathy and will-less resignation, is a state to which we may become subject though it is not characteristic of our essential nature. If this appears to be confusing consider the way we grow through life — a child may be constantly subject to impatience or be characteristically dreamy but will not have an innate disposition to despair. We are born in hope, it is only later when misfortune and adverse circumstances have laid us low that we are prey to hopelessness. In the same way it is only when the impatient child is constantly frustrated that anger or resentment may develop.

9

The 38 remedies were discovered by Bach by a combination of intuition and suffering. He was an extraordinarily sensitive man and having once recognised the condition that he sought to heal he was able to sense the appropriate remedy. Many of the states for which he later found an antidote he experienced in himself as an intense suffering both mental and physical. This personal suffering was to shorten his life, he died in 1936 at the age of 50, but it was a sure way to find the remedy that was needed.[1]

The remedies have been spoken of by name as flowers. In fact it is not the plant itself that represents the healing quality but the energy that is within the flower. This energy is extracted by most careful though simple methods. A thin glass bowl is taken and filled with pure water. Sufficient flowers are picked and floated on the water so as to cover the surface. This must be done on a clear sunny day when there are no clouds in the sky and the flowers are in perfect bloom. The bowl is then left in the sunlight for three to four hours or less time if the blooms show signs of fading. By a process of natural alchemy the healing energy within the flowers is transferred into the water. The flowers are then removed and the liquid is poured into bottles with an equal volume of brandy which acts as a preservative.

Some of the remedies, like *Chestnut Bud* and *Willow* cannot be prepared in this way and they are made by the 'boiling method'. With these remedies the selected parts of the plant are boiled for 30 minutes in pure water, strained off and the liquid preserved with brandy as in the 'sunshine method'. This extract from the plant is the 'essence'. Two drops of essence are sufficient to potentise a one ounce bottle of brandy — this is now 'stock' of that particular remedy. When a patient is treated two drops are taken from the stock bottle and placed in an ounce of water with a teaspoonful of brandy which again acts as a preservative; this is the medicine bottle from which the patient takes his dosage. In most cases a prescribed medicine consists of between one and five remedies put in together, two drops from each stock bottle. The patient then takes four drops of this four times a day for as long as required — usually a period of a few weeks, sometimes a couple of months. Prepared stocks of the different remedies can be obtained from the Dr Edward Bach Centre.

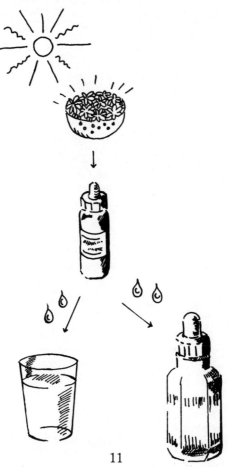

THE HEALING POWER
OF NATURE

One of the most striking features of this form of healing is that it is entirely benign. It involves no physical discomfort and is associated only with the most pure and beautiful elements in nature. With a few exceptions (*Vine, Olive* and *Cerato*) all the plants used grow wild and free without the taint of human interference. When Bach was first looking for the remedies he discounted any plants that were poisonous, cultivated or closely associated with man. He sought only those that were growing in the most natural conditions where their powerful healing properties had matured undisturbed and uncontaminated. We can readily recognise the importance of this feeling of strength and purity. It is apparent as soon as one sees the remedies: they have an aura of great lightness and clarity. Even the stock bottles themselves had a simple fitness and beauty that characterised all Dr Bach's work.

Conventional medicine, which today relies so heavily upon artificial drugs, points a strong contrast. The idea of preparing a chemical extract of the healing properties in natural substances is totally antipathetic to Bach's work. There is an extraordinary perversity in man when he deliberately seeks such complex methods of working and ignores the virtues of what is simple, natural and God-given. It is no coincidence that medicinal herbs are traditionally called 'simples'.

This is no place for a polemic against the artifice of modern life. But in the context of the Bach Remedies it is good to consider the relationship between disease and the healing power of nature. Man is "a child of the Universe no less than the trees and stars" and yet we live in daily conflict with the rest of the natural world. Much of the disease to which we are prey at this time is generated by this conflict, in particular the nervous conditions that are so prevalent in urban life. Anger and fear which in their broadest sense are two primary conditions that colour our psyche are both eased and healed by contact with the natural world. We need only consider the effect of a seaside holiday upon the oppressed city-dweller to see the reality of this. Irritation, tension, pride or depression are not cured by aspirins — they merely deaden the receptors of the nervous system. But the recognition of man's true relationship to the created world can attune the disharmony of our life and release us from our suffering.

The Bach Remedies, which contain the pure energies of the natural world, help us to tune our selves in this way. Yet their effect is not merely to soothe and calm the turbulence of our personalities. Through the action of specific energies they help us to tackle specific problems. The general impact of nature's healing power is not sufficient to counteract man's anger and greed; if it was we could not choose but to live harmoniously in this world. But by using the potentised energy from a particular flower, whose properties are exactly aligned to a particular condition, we have a concentration of that general healing power that can actually bring about a change within us so that hatred may become love, despair may find faith, indifference may become purposeful and the exhausted may find strength.

13

HOW THE REMEDIES WORK

In his book *Heal Thyself* Bach states that there are certain fundamental truths that have to be acknowledged if we are to understand the nature of disease:

1 That man has a Soul which is his Real Self. The body is the 'earthly temple' that the Soul inhabits though it is but a small reflection of the Soul itself. The Soul which is the immortal spark of our Divinity, a manifestation of the Almighty, is our guide and protector, the watcher who leads us always for our utmost advantage.

2 That our personality, through which we act in this world, is down here to gain experience and knowledge so that we may advance towards the perfection of our natures by developing virtues and eradicating that which is wrong within us.

3 That this life is but a small part of the whole process of our evolution, a day in the endless time that our Soul experiences as immortality.

4 That just so long as our Soul and personality are in harmony we live in peace, happiness, joy and health. It is when our

personality leads us astray from the path laid down for it by the Soul, either through worldly desire or through the persuasion of others, that conflict arises.

5 That there is Unity in all things. The One Creator who is Love manifests through innumerable forms and all things are unified by that Love. Any imperfection in a part affects the whole and every part of the whole must ultimately become perfect in Love.

6 The fundamental errors that bring conflict and then disease are dissociation between our Soul and personality and wrongdoing which is a sin against Unity.

This is only a précis of Bach's own statements concerning man's relationship to Creation and the Almighty. What he wrote, in turn, is but a brief outline of the great tradition of knowledge, wisdom and understanding that man has received by Grace concerning the nature of reality. Two points are of immediate concern to us here — that disease can be beneficent in that it points out to us the conflict that lies within us and that an essential part of the healing process is the work that we must do upon ourselves, the work of self-development. It is in this context that we should view the way that the Bach Remedies work.

Given that the remedies work upon the subtle world it is not surprising that conventional scientific thinking cannot be used to explain their operation. If we were to attempt a chemical analysis of a remedy we would not be able to detect the physical substance that is the healing agent. This is because it is not a physical substance. It is what may be best described as energy.

15

We have already seen that Dr Bach found it essential to consider man as being composed of different levels or bodies, of which the familiar physical body is the coarsest and the most dense. To express it very simply this physical body is animated and controlled by the Soul which acts through the psychological body. We may recognise the psychological body as the thoughts, feelings and emotions that together make up the pattern of our personality. The essential energy of life, which comes from a higher level, is 'filtered' through this pattern so that it is coloured by the condition of the psyche before it is drawn into the physical body. Thus the psychological state of an individual will set up certain energy vibrations that will register in the physical body. Consider, for instance, how irritation, a psychological state, may cause a person to frown. If this pattern is consistent over a period of time lines of irritation will develop into creases which permanently mark the face. Thus it is said that we make our own faces.

It this is not clear let us use an analogy. When a plant begins to grow it does so in a perfect and uniform way. The first leaves and shoots are identical in every plant of that species. But the prevailing conditions will slowly distort and condition that growth into a form which in time becomes characteristic of that individual. One tree is exposed to a westerly wind off the sea which bends it into a particular shape; another which grows beside a wall may become lopsided and misshapen. In both cases the tree is at variance with the balanced growth that would be seen in the 'perfect image' of that type of tree.

So it is with human beings. The patterning of our psychological condition sets up a rhythm in the body that can distort its normal workings. A tree cannot reshape itself but it is possible for a man to actively change his physical condition by

16

changing the psychological patterning of his life. If a person who has been constantly fearful is able to be free from that fear it has a very real and observable effect upon the physical body. The Bach Remedies can be instrumental in bringing about this change. If we suppose that every psychological state, as they are described by Bach, has a particular pattern to it and that the pattern acts as a distorting lens to the pure light that shines through from the Soul of man, then the remedies act upon that pattern to dissolve the distortion and allow the free passage of clear energy to the body.

This psychological pattern might also be thought of as an oscillating wave with regular peaks and troughs. The remedy that is its antidote would then be seen to have a wave pattern that was exactly opposite, so that the two put together produce a harmonious and balanced condition. Or to use another illustration the psychological pattern might be seen as colours. Then the make up of an individual psyche would appear as a combination of different hues that surround the body as a aura — a vibrating force field of colour. We know from the expression 'it made me see red' how anger would affect such a pattern. Similarly we speak of people 'green with envy' or 'grey with fear'. In each case there is a Bach Remedy that would be appropriate. *Holly* for anger and envy (red and green are complimentaries) and *Rock Rose* for extreme fear. As the healing energy of the remedy worked upon the psyche the grey clouds of fear would be dispersed by the radiating sun of courage and joy which allows all things to be seen in their true light. But should the fits of anger be allowed to continue without any check then not only would their red colour the entire psyche, they would in time produce such a permanent distortion in the flow of the life force that the physical body would be damaged as extensively as if exposed to prolonged radiation.

At this point it is as well to note that the remedies are very beneficial when used to prevent illness, to balance the psyche before the disruption goes so far as to produce a recognisable physical complaint. For even a temporary condition can debilitate the body to such an extent that it is susceptible to those forces of disease that are constantly present in the environment. Virus infections, for instance, only take hold in the body when the normal defences are weakened. Thus when we are in a state of indecision (*Scleranthus*) or are undecided what to do in life (*Wild Oat*) we are prone to suffer from the mundane illnesses that afflict most people from time to time.

It will be appreciated that a minor affliction will be healed more quickly and more readily than a deep-rooted condition. Disease, pain and suffering develop like an organic growth fed from the psychological state. If for instance we consider the remedy *Beech* which is appropriate to the critical, fussy, intolerant person who gets annoyed by the habits and mannerisms of others, then we can see that every time that person makes a criticism they add another branch to the tree of their own suffering. Every time they have a negative thought another leaf unfolds until the growth of the tree presses so sorely upon them that they are forced to recognise their own condition. Their suffering will in time bring them to ask the question "Why?".

Often enough we refuse to see the link between our psychological outlook and our physical suffering. We may gain temporary relief from some form of medication but if the real cause if not recognised and eliminated then the suffering will inevitably return. This is one reason

18

why drugs are often counterproductive: they give the appearance of a rapid return to normality when the cause of the ill health is as virulent as ever. We are lulled into a false sense of well-being and continue in the pattern that must result in more serious consequences.

It is important for us to recognise the link between our psychological state and our physical complaint. By recognising the situation we are able to work with the remedy and hasten the change within ourselves. It is not an imperative part of the treatment, however. The Bach Remedies have been used with proven success in the treatment of children, animals and plants. Self-awareness is not a precondition for a cure.

It was said earlier that disease is beneficial since it points to the need for self-development and the resolution of internal conflict. It is as if the Bach Remedies show us the way in which we have to work upon ourselves and help us to overcome the habitual psychological patterns that have developed within us. If we want to return to health we must expect to change. Many of us are resistant to change; we have almost grown to like our suffering and secretly prefer to indulge in our unhappiness (there is a remedy for that too). Sometimes there is an unwillingness to acknowledge a psychological imbalance — we insist that the malady is purely physical and do not want anything that may tamper with the personality: the ego works hard to protect its little empire! As it is said, you can take a horse to water but you cannot make it drink — nothing can be done if you do not take the medicine. As with all forms of healing it is important that the patient should want to improve his condition.

WHEN WE TAKE A REMEDY

Although the action of the remedies is entirely benign it is not possible to exactly predict the course of their action. In many cases the patient will feel no immediate effect. Sometimes there is a sense of relief and well-being, we may feel the tension ease and so be able to observe the action of the remedy. Occasionally the patient is abruptly faced by the real nature of his personality which may be a surprising confrontation. It depends to some extent upon the sensitivity and state of the patient. There are many case histories which record a startling improvement in the illness. When dealing with an hysterical person or one who is unconscious we can expect an immediate response while a chronic condition may shift quite slowly. Since we cannot quantify a psychological state, it is a matter of quality not quantity, it is not possible to systematically predict results. Thus we do not prescribe a seven-day course as with antibiotics but deal entirely on an individual basis with the needs of the patient.

Treating the patient individually is important since it is sometimes necessary to change the remedy as the psychological condition changes. As we come to face the reality of our situation it is possible that new conflicts may arise. In the first stages there may be a clear improvement and then perhaps a setback, the patient feels discouraged and doubts that he will ever be really well. At such a point it is very clear that an additional remedy is required — *Gentian*. This is for doubt and discouragement, a lack of faith and conviction. So the new psychological condition is tackled and resolved.

Just as the suffering of the patient has grown organically like a tree that puts out a new branch each time the diseased pattern of behaviour is confirmed, so too it is dismembered branch by branch. Sometimes it is necessary to trace back the psychological condition through many states, using first one remedy and then another. Thus we slowly cut back to the root of the problem and properly eradicate the cause of the imbalance. The physical body will gradually improve during this process until it is fully well. It is a naturally self-righting mechanism and when no longer subject to the stress and imbalance of the psyche it should automatically adjust its functions to good working order.

It would be improper to suggest that every disease can be treated with equal success. As with all healing there are some patients who cannot be cured. This may be owing to a pathological state that is beyond recall or where an organ has been permanently damaged; there may be an overriding condition that prevents the patient being healed; it may be that at the Soul level the subject knows that it is right for the illness to continue, or there is an inborn defect in the physical body which is beyond the scope of the Bach Remedies to deal with.

So while the remedies will help to deal with the psychological condition the state of the body may not be automatically 'cured'. It may be appropriate, therefore, to work in conjunction with other techniques such as osteopathy or Alexander method which would work to re-align the body and its energy systems or with surgery when there is extreme physical damage. In the latter case the remedies are very useful to deal with the shock and distress involved. In every situation the Bach Remedies can be helpful since the number of people whose psyche is properly balanced are few indeed.

It should be remembered that true healing is not just the action of removing the physical suffering but also helping the patient to come to terms with the significance of the illness. This brings us to the way in which the remedies can be used as a means of self-development. Although this is not within the bounds of normal medical interest it is an integral part of the process of health. For the most part we only treat with sickness and pay little attention to the subject of health. We have seen that physical illness is directly related to a decline in psychological health. It is a law of existence that it is impossible to remain stationary. That which is not making forward progress must be in decline — everything is either in the process of growing or in the process of dying. So it is with our own psychological state: if we are not making forward progress in self-development then we are literally on the way to ill health. Therefore we each have a responsibility to ourselves to work at the psychological level to improve the condition of our lives. Bach refers to this in terms of the perfection of our nature and the development of virtues.

The Bach Remedies then can be used directly as a form of psychological therapy, not just for those who are recognised as being mentally sick but for all people. To make the point again, there are very few people whose psyche is perfectly balanced. Using the remedies in this way may often be a process of 'self-encounter'. We must first face the reality of our personality and see what sort of person we are. It may be unpleasant for the ego to acknowledge that it is wilful, inflexible, possessive or proud. Other people can see these traits but we are rarely willing to acknowledge them ourselves. Then it may be necessary to face up to emotions and feelings that we have repressed and come to terms with past situations that we prefer to keep locked away in the deeper recesses of the memory. Taking a remedy may bring many things to the surface for consideration. It is as if the psyche were a river and on this river float many logs, the memories that are constantly being taken from the external world and thrown into the waters of the mind. Normally they float downstream to the sawmill as the useful material of experience for building the structure of our life. But log-jams can occur and although the water flows on we are not making use of the lessons that are daily being shown to us. An appropriate remedy can then help us to walk out on to the river to free the logs and so set in motion again the proper flow of the psyche.

When such a situation occurs much productive work can be done by the individual. In the long run it is extremely beneficial though it can occasionally be unsettling at the time, if only because we may have a succession of vivid dreams as the logs go down river. However, this does not constitute a 'healing crisis' and we may be able to come to terms with ourselves without any conflict or upset. Certainly it should be made clear that psychological disturbance is not an inevitable side effect. The response is dependent upon why we take the remedy. If we choose to work in this way then the remedy will not work with us. If the intention is not in this direction then it will not have this effect. The individual is always in control, it is not like taking drugs which upset the psychological metabolism through interference. The remedies cooperate with our guide and internal teacher, the Soul, who, as Bach said, works always for our utmost advantage.

DIAGNOSIS AND
PRESCRIBING

Most systems of medicine require long training in a complex methodology both for the diagnosis and treatment. It is a very remarkable feature of the Bach Remedies that not only is the method of treatment extremely simple but that the diagnosis is also very straightforward, once the essentials of the system have been grasped. This means that it is possible to treat yourself, thus obviating the need for a professional practitioner. Bach entitled his book 'Heal Thyself'. It may be that in the first instance we go to a Bach practitioner, somebody with experience, who can explain the system and diagnose the condition more readily. But in many cases a patient soon obtains their own set of remedies, treats themselves and then subsequently perhaps they can provide remedies for others, their family and friends. The time may come when the Bach Remedies are found in every home as an integral part of the medicine chest.

All that is needed in order to prescribe is a clear perception of the psychological condition of the person. This is not a technical matter, it is common sense. The very experience of life qualifies us to see what is needed. It does not require a university degree to recognise fear, anger, resentment or lack of confidence: they are self-evident. So we can be sure that any adult who is reasonably aware of human nature is qualified to practice. Since there can be no ill effects from a wrong diagnosis the system has a built-in safety mechanism which guards against mishap. If we choose the wrong remedy we simply do not heal the psychological problem. Experience brings accuracy and accuracy speeds the healing process in every medical discipline.

The Twelve Healers and Other Remedies

Bach named the first twelve remedies that he discovered *The Twelve Healers*. Later he found another 26 so that in all there are 38 remedies that are applicable as either type remedies or helping remedies. More comprehensive information is given in other books (see p. 51) but it should be possible to recognise the broad qualities from the following list.

For Fear

Rock Rose *for emergencies, sudden illness or accident, for very great fear, terror, panic, hysteria, when life is despaired of, for the horror and dread of nightmares, when there has been a close encounter with evil. Symptoms may include paralysis, unconsciousness, suddenly dumb/deaf, icy coldness, trembling, loss of control.*

Mimulus *fear of worldly, physical things like animals, heights, pain, accidents, of water, the dark, of illness, death, being alone, of other people, stage fright, any specific fear of known origin but often indisclosed. Symptoms may include stuttering, blushing, sinus trouble (running nose/eyes), shallow breathing, marked sensitivity to noise, controversy and crowds; nervous disposition, shyness.*

26

Cherry Plum *for desperation, fear of insanity, loss of control, an uncontrollable impulse, nervous breakdown, suicidal, obsessive fear, delusions. Symptoms usually build up over a period of time: pallor, staring eyes, agitation, sometimes nervous talk or obsessive questioning, imminent mild insanity. It is like mental gangrene, very offensive to the self.*

Aspen *for psychological fears of unknown origin, vague unreasoning and inexplicable, sudden apprehension, fear of unseen power or force, fear of sleep for fear of what will come, fear from dreams, association with death and religion, usually kept secret. Symptoms may include headaches, eyestrain, haunted look, sweating, trembling, gooseflesh, sudden faintness, sleep walking/talking, tired and nervy.*

Red Chestnut *for those who find it difficult not to be anxious for other people, anticipate trouble, imagine the worst, worry over others' troubles, overconcern for problems of the world, fear that a small complaint from another will become a serious problem, project anxiety.*

For Uncertainty

Cerato *people doubt their own abilities, they are weak-willed and lack courage of their conviction, distrust self and always ask other's advice, distrust own intuition and judgement, often foolish, changeable, imitative, easily led astray. They are often talkative, asking many questions, often rejected by peer group as a child, a follower.*

Scleranthus *people cannot make up their minds, cannot choose between two things, changeable and indecisive, lack concentration, hesitant, unstable, and tend to be unreliable. They are quiet and do not seek advice, suffer extremes of energy, joy/sadness and cannot handle the alternating moods. Recognisable by lack of balance and* poise, erratic conversation, hesitancy, restlessness, always different clothes, changeable outlook, symptoms move about, come and go, liable to travel sickness.

Gentian for those who are easily discouraged, get depressed and disheartened, for doubt and lack of faith, for melancholy, scepticism and disappointment. Depression from a known cause, from delay or hindrance and the distress caused by a temporary setback in progress, for the negativity that breeds a sense of failure. Indicated by a pervasive gloom and sadness.

Gorse for despair, great hopelessness, chronic depression and resignation, loss of will to improve conditions. Believe that nothing can be done to help though may be persuaded to try again whilst thinking it futile, needs to be pushed — Gorse heals the inner will. Symptoms may be a condition that apparently cannot be cured, a genetic illness, repeated failure or disappointment. Often seen with dark rings under eyes, hopeless expression, just sits, inert, hopeless beyond tears or expression of grief, complexion may be sallow in developed state.

Hornbeam for a temporary state of mental/ physical tiredness when a lack of energy causes loss of interest, weariness and inability to cope with mundane affairs. Good for convalescents who feel unable to return to work through perfectly fit. Symptoms are predominant fatigue, lassitude, inclination to lie in bed in mornings, feel they cannot face the burden of the day.

Wild Oat for uncertainty with regard to career (a cause of more problems than is realised) indefinite/ unfulfilled ambition, drifters who allow ambition to fade, often talented but unable to follow one occupation that is their real calling. Symptoms may include despondency, general dissatisfaction and uncertainty, feeling of frustration, boredom, often find themselves in uncongenial environments and occupations.

28

Insufficient Interest in Present Circumstances

Clematis *people are dreamers, absent-minded, lack concentration and vitality, quiet people without proper interest in present, absorbed in thoughts and fantasy, sleepy and unobservant, romantic, imaginative, unrealistic. Symptoms may include drowsiness, constant inclination to sleep, distant drifting feeling, marked pallor, slowness, sensitivity to noise, numbness, faintness, indifference, make little effort to get well and may even welcome prospect of death, often stumbling, drop things through inattention, 'float off' in conversation, lackadaisical air.*

Honeysuckle *for nostalgia, homesickness, those who live much in the past, past loves, happiness, unhappiness, regrets, success or failures, those who live on their memories, desiring to escape present in romanticised view of past.*

Wild Rose *for resignation, apathy, surrender, failure to make effort, fatalism, just drift down hill, dullness, lack of interest, no spark or vitality, sense of monotony, expressionless drone to voice, weariness, dull companion.*

Olive *for those who suffer from complete mental/ physical exhaustion, who have drained their reserves of energy so that they have no more strength. Applicable after prolonged illness, lengthy sickbed nursing, a personal ordeal (war, divorce, crisis etc.) after long overwork or over-worry, when a superhuman effort has been made. When we are mentally and physically rundown.*

White Chestnut *for a pattern of thoughts that constantly repeats and gives no rest to the mind, continual internal argument, worry and chatter, mental congestion. Thoughts circulate without resolution, going over and over the same conflict, preoccupation that obstructs clarity, a drama is forever re-enacted in the mind and gives no rest. Symptoms*

29

may include tiredness, insomnia, confusion, depression, guilt feelings, repetition of a topic in conversation, lack of calmness, nervous worry, often causes headaches.

Mustard for depression that comes for no apparent reason from an unknown cause, gloom, deep sadness, melancholy, usually serious people who feel that they suffer periodic affliction from a malefic star. Depression is intense and cannot be alleviated until it lifts as unexpectedly as it came. All joy and peace is driven out of life for the duration.

Chestnut Bud for those who fail to learn by experience and go on repeating the same mistakes again and again. They may be impatient and always thinking ahead and so fail to see what is happening, failing to base their actions upon past experience. They may be careless, clumsy, slow in learning, inattentive and as children even apparently retarded.

For Loneliness

Water Violet for those who like to be alone, they are aloof sometimes proud, quiet and retiring, avoid argument, self-relaint, inward-looking, very capable, peaceful and calming. They are self-contained people who know their own minds, may appear disdainful and condescending, they are tolerant and never interfere in the affairs of others, just as they will not tolerate interference. They bear their grief and sorrows in silence. They may suffer from physical rigidity, stiffness and tension since their energy is often blocked.

Impatiens for those impatient people who dislike restraint, preferring to work alone at their own speed, they like haste in all things, are critical of others' shortcomings, irritable, impulsive, impetuous, active and intelligent though prone to nervous tension, overexertion and accidents.

Symptoms may include sudden pains, cramps, tension in back, neck, jaws, hands, shoulders, indigestion. Children may be irritable and demanding. Body often slopes forward, they lead, going ahead and act quickly, will finish sentence for other people who think more slowly. Given to outbursts of temper though it quickly subsides.

Heather people are greedy for the attention of others, very talkative, compulsively discuss their affairs with anyone, cannot bear to be alone, fearful people who seek sympathy and live on the energy of others. They are self-centred and overconcerned with their own lives and problems. Recognisable by the constant chatter, stand close to you, it is difficult to get away, lack of interest in other people, bad listeners, hypochondriacs (to get attention).

Oversensitive to Ideas and Influences

Agrimony appears cheerful, jovial and uncomplaining but hides mental torture and worry behind a carefree mask. Restless, seeks excitement and activity to overcome worry, often takes drugs or alcohol to forget self and dull pain and suffering. Peace loving, avoid quarrels and argument, hide sensitivity but restless and nervy. Will often not admit to problems when asked and when ill will joke and make light of the matter.

Centaury people are timid, quiet, kind, gentle, conventional and anxious to please, weak-willed, docile and easily dominated so that in helping others they become a servile drudge. They are often bound to a more forceful personality who exploits their good nature though they choose such situations since they are submissive and seek strength of personality in others rather than in themselves. Symptoms may affect shoulders and back (burdens), white faced with rings under eyes, languid, sits bowed.

31

Walnut *for those who need protection from outside influences when foundation of life is unsettled during a major change in life — teething, puberty, starting a new school/career/job, any fundamental alteration in mental, emotional or physical state. Helps to break with the old and establish pattern of new. Guards against anything that interferes with workings of normal life, protects those who are attacked by subtle forces, known as the 'link breaker'.*

Holly *for any kind of strongly negative state: anger, jealousy, bitterness, envy, rage, suspicion, revenge, hatred, violence, bad temper, contempt, vexation, selfishness, frustration — all states which are antipathetic to love.*

For Despondency and Despair

Larch *for those who lack confidence in themselves, they expect failure and feel they will never succeed and so do not try hard enough, they are hesitant and procrastinate, succumb easily and feel inferior. Their sense of failure makes them despondent thought in fact they are perfectly capable if they could persevere. Symptoms may include general depression and is often associated with impotence.*

Pine *is for self-reproach, guilt, those who blame themselves, self-condemnation, often assuming responsibility for a situation that is not their fault. They are discontented and critical of themselves, overconscientious, apologetic and over-humble. The constant effort they make to improve themselves may lead to tiredness and depression. Helps to alleviate any feelings of guilt.*

Elm *for those who are very capable and often carry great responsibility but occasionally feel unable to face the magnitude of their tasks. Thus they are sometimes overwhelmed, falter and momentarily lose confidence. It is as if they have temporarily* lost their connection and this causes great discomfort and distress.

Sweet Chestnut *for a time of terrible anguish and despair when we are at the uttermost limits of endurance, there appears to be no light or love left in our world, nothing but destruction and annihilation, utter desolation, unable even to pray, the 'dark night of the soul'.*

Star of Bethlehem *for shock, grief, distress, for those who need consolation and comfort, for bad news, an accident, fright, a narrow escape, for delayed shock, to neutralise effects of any shock past or present, even the shock of birth.*

Willow *for those who suffer any small adversity with bitterness and resentment, they blame others and feel hard done by, they are self-centred, self-pitying, self-justifying, feel wronged, sulk and bear grudges, will feel slighted and constantly dissatisfied, lack humour. Symptoms may include constant frowning, grumbling, spread a gloom and feeling of negativity, a difficult patient since nothing pleases and reluctance to admit improvement.*

Oak *strong, reliable, patient, responsible people who shoulder great burdens without complaint. They are plodders who persevere inspite of setbacks, never giving up hope. Their unceasing efforts and obstinacy may led to exhaustion and owing to their willingness to take on more than they can manage and then keep going through all difficulties they can eventually come to a point of breakdown. Ill health causes dissatisfaction and despondency since it brings limitation. For those who never stop trying however hopeless their situation.*

Crab Apple *the cleansing remedy, for those who feel in some way unclean, contaminated, often minor ailment that assumes great importance in the mind of the sufferer causing despondency and self-disgust. Applicable to physical or psychological* condition, wherever there is something repellent to the self, the remedy restores a sense of proportion. Symptoms may include skin ailments, poison in body or a wound, unwholesome habits, smelly feet, dislike of physical contact e.g. breast-feeding.

Overcare for Welfare of Others

Chicory *for people who can be most truly loving but when in a negative state become possessive, their egotism, self-pity/self-love makes them over-concerned about their relationship to others. They can become critical, fussy, bossy, correcting, toxic with mental/emotional poisons, seek attention, tearful and thwarted, dislike being alone and need to have their loved ones near in order to control and direct their activity. Recognisable as 'mothering type' through prevalent in children who demand attention.*

Vervain *people are forceful, enthusiastic, overbearing, highly strung, argumentative, directing, fervent, fanatical, they rarely change their fixed opinions and insist that others should be converted to them. They have strong will and can exhaust themselves through over-effort. Symptoms may include physical tension, muscle strain, headaches, eyestrain, forceful expression, over-activity, inability to relax.*

Vine *capable people who are certain of themselves and tend to use their authority to gain power and dominate others. May be arrogant, ambitious, bossy, exacting, rigid, strict, lacking in sympathy, violent, cruel, demand obedience. They are leaders who while they may be of great value in emergency tend to be ruthless in obtaining their own ends, can be tyrants and dictators. Tends to heavy chest development, big stature, often suffer from extreme tension, physical stiffness, back problems, high blood pressure.*

Beech *for those who are critical, dissatisfied, intolerant, irritable, always finding fault, seeing only the negative side of things. Annoyed by small matters — the oddities, mannerisms and idiosyncrasies of others; demand exactness, order and discipline. Arrogant people who complain of others, petty anger, sound in judgement but sour, cynical, unsympathetic, strict with others, tense. Tends to affect upper chest areas, tension in jaws, arms and hands from clenching.*

Rock Water *very strict people who deny themselves, self-repressed, ruled by theories and rigid through strong conviction of what is 'right'. Greedy for perfection but trapped by trying too hard, idealists who cannot see the obsession which dominates them. Prone to fanaticism and spiritual pride, wish to be a shining example to others. Often relates to a food fetish, those overconcerned with diet, purity of living, strict morality, wherever a too rigid self discipline may cause suffering.*

Recognising the Remedy

Let us assume that we are to prescribe for a patient Mrs X. She is a neighbour who has suffered for many years with migraine and rheumatism, she wakes early in the morning and then with the physical discomfort she is unable to get back to sleep. She is a forceful personality who is always trying to get things done locally, she constantly has a battle on hand: getting the local council to sweep the street more regularly, fighting a demolition order on the old church, trying to stop the lorries from taking a short cut down past her house and so on. Every time you meet her you are asked to sign another petition. She is really not well but still keeps going, organising and agitating for the things that she feels are important and right. Mrs X gets very angry when her campaigns are not successful and bitter about the failure of the local people to support her cause. Then she gets a migraine. But instead of giving up she simply sets to again with renewed effort refusing to accept defeat.

First we must try to recognise the type remedy for such a person. It will be quickly apparent that *Vervain* is most applicable — it equates with her strong opinions and forceful, almost fanatical zeal for her cause that is felt to be right. *Holly* would be appropriate to the anger and if we probe more deeply we might find that other remedies suggest themselves — *Willow* for the resentment and sense of failure when the campaign has not been successful and the sense of injustice that she suffers, *Beech* might be needed to counteract the tendency to see only those things that are wrong in her life and her intolerance of every small imperfection in the society in which she lives. Since this is a fictitious case we are only intent upon seeing the sort of remedies that would be indicated.

Mrs X will always be an enthusiastic type of person but with a course of Bach Remedies it is possible for her to channel that energy in a positive and creative way, eliminating the negative effects which have caused her physical suffering. The positive side of her personality will then manifest in a more tolerant and broad-minded approach to the problems of life which in the long run is likely to achieve far more than the forceful 'head-on' approach used previously.

We may see from such an example how the choice of remedies is usually self-evident. It is not necessary for a person to demonstrate every aspect of a particular remedy for it to be appropriate. We always look for the general tendency. Often this can be recognised in an odd phrase or a particular emphasis given to one attitude. It is usually possible to diagnose by just listening to a person's remarks about themselves. The following statements, for instance, would each give a clear indication of an appropriate remedy.

1 "I am so critical of everyone and everything — I cannot see any good points in anyone at present."

2 "He is impossible just now, insists we always do as he wants, as he is always right, lays down the law and is so stern with the children they are quite frightened of him."

3 "I feel like nothing on earth, exhausted and weak and have no interest in anything."

4 "I am almost tortured by feelings of insecurity."

5 "It is no use, I have tried so many things."

6 "Mentally she wears a hair shirt, ruling herself with a rod of iron."

7 "She did not see me when I passed her in the street. She was far away in her thoughts."

8 "I cannot keep my mind on what I am doing — all kinds of other thoughts keep crowding in."

9 "I make the same mistake time after time."

10 "I have asked advice from so many people and acted on it but it has never been satisfactory."

In order these statements would indicate the following remedies:

1	Beech	6	Rock Water
2	Vine	7	Clematis
3	Olive	8	White Chestnut
4	Mimulus	9	Chestnut Bud
5	Gorse	10	Cerato

Any attitude that is expressed in this way can be used to pinpoint the remedy that should be used. It may be helpful to discover the patient's attitude (or our own) towards certain general areas of activity. Do you find decision making difficult? If you constantly ask advice *Cerato* is indicated. If you cannot make up your mind — *Scleranthus*; you cannot decide what occupation to follow? — *Wild Oat*. Then again how do you feel about working with a group of people? If you are fearful — *Mimulus*; prefer to work alone — *Water Violet*; find others too slow — *Impatiens*; always dominate the group — *Vine*; end up as the dog's body — *Centaury*; enjoy groups because you can always find somebody to talk to — *Heather*; the list could go on.

Often the physical aspect will give an immediate indication. Perhaps the person just looks dreamy and so it is easy to recognise the *Clematis* state. Sometimes we may suspect a type remedy, *Impatiens*, for instance, but then have to check that it is right. Ask about the approach to work: if they are slow and thorough then it is unlikely to be *Impatiens*. If they are rather slapdash and in a hurry to get the job finished then we are on the right track. Then check by considering the way they walk (fast, tense, always in front) and then perhaps the way they react to criticism. Every response will bring a clearer picture of the personality concerned.

As experience is gained in working with the remedies a background of understanding is developed. Apart from recognising the specific nature of each remedy we can anticipate the circumstances that will be likely to indicate a particular state and can then also help with supportive counselling. We have mentioned the use of *Gentian* to overcome a temporary setback in an illness. Similarly *Centaury* is often helpful for old people who have given up in the face of difficulties. *Honeysuckle* is also good for old age, especially when there has been a bereavement, it helps when we find it difficult to carry on after a loved one has gone. It is helpful whenever there is a parting of the ways.

Red Chestnut is needed for over-anxious mums and also helps those who work in hospitals or in situations when subjective involvement may bring overconcern for others. *White Chestnut* may also be coupled with *Red Chestnut* when we cannot stop the worrying thoughts. *Mimulus* should be taken when we know that we have to undergo an ordeal or initiation that is causing anxiety, it is helpful for old people afraid of dying. *Rock Rose* is helpful for those about to go into battle, it brings courage and fortitude, enabling us to forget ourselves. Take it before going to the dentist — that too may call for courage.

Cherry Plum, Gorse and *Sweet Chestnut* are three remedies that tackle extremes of depression and despair. We may suffer from such a condition at any age but it is well to remember that a *Cherry Plum* state sometimes affects young people — the great distress of adolescent depression. *Cherry Plum* is also applicable when treating with the disturbance caused by drug reaction. It may be appropriate to combine it with *Clematis* when the patient is not properly 'earthed'. *Clematis* should be given for any kind of fainting, coma, unconsciousness and the feelings that come before and afterwards — when you are just lightheaded.

Depression is not easily dealt with by a reasoning approach, by its nature it is often irrational — here the Bach Remedies are particularly helpful. *Mustard* or *Gentian* are usually appropriate; *Gentian* when we know why we are depressed, *Mustard* when the cause is unknown.

It is important to realise how to be supportive to a person so as to encourage their strengths and strengthen their weakness. Remember that every remedy has a positive as well as a negative expression, it is by developing the positive expression that a person fulfils his real nature. We

should always work with sympathy and understanding using the power of love that comes
from the heart, not just the head. In this way we
will perceive how it is appropriate to approach
and then where relevant to assist each individual. With an *Agrimony* type, for instance, it is
unwise to probe too deeply, they are best persuaded by kindness and a gentle understanding.
With an *Aspen* state it is well to direct the attention towards earthing activities where a physical
contact is made as through gardening, bread-
making, pottery etc. Such ideas can be intro-
duced without force, by gentle suggestion. For
an *Olive* condition sleep is a great healer. Where
Sweet Chestnut is indicated so is fresh air and
sunlight and a contact with nature. As before the
list could continue but this is sufficient to indicate
a relationship between the different remedies
and the different ways of working that each may
require.

Sometimes it is difficult to settle upon a clear
diagnosis. Either we seem to need all the
remedies or none of them appears that clearly
indicated. Alternatively it may happen that a
treatment reaches an impasse and there is no
further improvement. In such circumstances
there are three remedies that act as catalysts,
working to shift the operation so that the condition may be clearly recognised. These catalysts
are *Holly, Wild Oat* and *Star of Bethlehem. Holly*
is best for the active type, *Wild Oat* for the
passive. *Star of Bethlehem* may be used to
counteract shock at any level, even though it
may be from years gone by and not even consciously remembered. That shock may be the
one log that jams the flow of the whole river.

Diagnosing for plants and animals is essen-
tially the same as diagnosing for people. We look
for the quality of the prime psychological state —
that is to say what does the plant or animal feel

40

like? A dog may be *Heather* type, always fussing about and telling you his problems; it may be a *Chicory* dog, always wanting to be on top of you and demanding attention. Cats are often *Water Violet* or if nervous may need *Mimulus*. It is the same with plants: some of them may need *Scleranthus*: they just cannot make up their mind. *Hornbeam* is good for weak or drooping plants. When afflicted with greenfly or mould they need *Crab Apple* to cleanse the infection and *Agrimony* for the torture that cannot be expressed. Like all living things they suffer from shock, fear, discouragement and hopelessness.

Combination Remedies

A particular combination of remedies has been found useful for seeds and seedling plants.[2] It is denoted by its initial letters HOV: *Hornbeam, Olive* and *Vine*. The *Vine* is to break down the hard shell of the seed, the *Hornbeam* gives strength and encourages the effort of development and the *Olive* overcomes the exhaustion that comes with the rapid expansion of germination and growth. Put one or two drops of each remedy into the can when watering.

Combination remedies are useful in other circumstances. A group of five remedies may be appropriate for those taking exams: it consists of *Gentian, Elm, Clematis, Larch* and *White Chestnut. Gentian* is for doubt and discouragement, *Elm* for the momentary loss of confidence, *Clematis* for the dreamy state that often occurs. *Larch* for the feeling of inadequacy and inability to succeed, *White Chestnut* helps concentration. Such a remedy works upon the positive will to succeed and so there is unlikely to be the usual anxiety and fears that exams can induce.

The most important combination remedy was

named by Bach as the *Rescue Remedy*. This consists of *Cherry Plum* for loss of control, *Clematis* for unconsciousness, *Impatiens* for stress, *Rock Rose* for terror and *Star of Bethlehem* for shock. *Rescue Remedy* is so useful for any situation major or minor that it is wise to have it prepared and on hand for emergencies. If it is taken immediately when an accident occurs, when we have bad news, when we are in any distress, even if we just have a headache it is very beneficial. Countless cases could be cited when *Rescue Remedy* has been used to overcome all manner of conditions.[4] It is also prepared as an ointment and may be applied to bruises and any damaged or inflamed skin condition. *Rescue Remedy* is so important that it is worth quoting a couple of instances of how it has worked.

Dr Bach used this combination first when he went to the aid of two men who were shipwrecked off the Cromer shore in a gale. It was many hours before the lifeboat got to them and they survived by roping themselves to the mast of the stricken boat. One man was unconscious when they reached the land, blue with cold and exhaustion. Dr Bach ran into the sea as they came ashore and moistened the man's lips with *Rescue Remedy*. He quickly recovered consciousness and a few minutes later sat up and asked for a cigarette. Another instance tells how a cook upset a frying pan of oil and burned her hand. She was running round the kitchen in shock and distress. When given *Rescue Remedy* (both drops and ointment) she became calm immediately and three hours later there was no pain, no blisters or even marks on the hand. A doctor quotes this use of *Rescue Remedy* for a middle-age man who had very low blood pressure after a heart attack, he was on an intravenous drip and in a very dangerous state. The *Rescue Remedy* was administered into the drip and the patient improved the next day and never looked back.

Dowsing

Some people have the ability to determine the appropriate remedy for a patient by means of various techniques of dowsing. In cases where this process is accurate it is of course an extremely effective way of prescribing. It must be stated, however, that the expertise of the practitioner is crucial — it is always important to be accurate in diagnosis and unless the accuracy is certain and can be validated by the results of treatment this form of diagnosis sets up an unnecessary complication. It prompts the question of why we should choose to work blind when it is so easy to see.

However, having made those qualifying remarks it may be helpful to see how dowsing techniques are used to diagnose and when they may be particularly useful. The sensivity of the dowser varies. Some people can simply hold an image of the patient in mind, run a finger over a list of remedies or the stock bottles and detect which remedies are required. This is sometimes registered as a direct cognition, sometimes a tingling sensation, a sharp 'electric' shock in the finger, even a sudden hiccup. Other people use a pendulum and with a prearranged signal for 'yes' and 'no' can detect the right remedies. Sometimes a witness is necessary, a photograph of the patient, a lock of hair or similar. If the patient is present it is possible, by holding their hand and then touching each remedy in turn, to gain a response from those that are needed.

On the face of it these methods would all be quick and efficient. If we have the real skill to dowse accurately we can detect a trait that might

43

be difficult to diagnose in a more normal way. If we are stuck and cannot find a remedy we might find it helpful to use a pendulum. But it is felt that a thorough knowledge of the remedies is more useful in the long run since it is then possible to employ all the skills of human endeavour to help the patient, not merely hand over the remedy trusting that it will do the trick. In most cases it is helpful to explain to the patient why a remedy is appropriate so that they may understand what their problem is and consciously work upon it. If we know the remedies well enough to be able to do that it is not usually necessary to resort to dowsing.

Some practitioners of radiesthenic techniques employ the principle of the Bach Remedies in treatment by transmitting the 'frequency' of a particular remedy to the patient. This does not involve taking the actual physical liquid of the remedy but the patient receives the same benefits as though he had taken it since the healing vibration is received directly by the subtle body. When such techniques are used the stock bottle or the name of the remedy is placed in a special relationship to the witness, perhaps by means of a particular healing pattern. Some healers can project the quality of a remedy without any tools and equipment and while such procedures stray beyond the scope of ordinary practice let us note one thing. If in an emergency we have the remedies with us then well and good. But should we be without their physical form we can actually call upon their help by concentrating intently upon their specific healing properties. If we can understand the subtle nature of the way that the remedies work then it should not be foreign to us to work in this way. Just as there is healing power in the essence of the flowers so too there is healing power in thought.

LEARNING TO DIAGNOSE

Leaving aside the somewhat imponderable procedures of dowsing let us look at the way in which we can effectively learn to diagnose by learning about the remedies themselves. When first faced by the 38 remedies there may seem to be a lot to take in. But a little careful study and observation makes the matter clear. The remedies represent what may be described as the archetypal conditions of humanity. So if we look we can quickly recognise people and situations which embody one or more remedies. This is very useful practice for those who wish to learn.

Consider the character of fairy stories. Many of them represent a type that is equivalent to a certain remedy. Cinderella, for instance, was a *Centaury*: she stayed at home dominated by the rest of the family, too weak-willed to stand up to them. For all her suffering though she was never resentful — she did not need *Willow*. Her sisters and stepmother needed a dose of *Vine* and *Holly* for they were tyrants and cruel taskmasters, the *Holly* might have helped them overcome their vexation when Cinderella was married to the charming Prince. Sleeping Beauty, of course, was badly in need of *Clematis*. And so we might suppose was Rip van Winkle and for him some *Star of Bethlehem* might have been in order.

Jack was a *Wild Oat* case until his Beanstalk offered him a ladder to fulfilment.

Looking at less romantic characters we could practise by prescribing for the characters in your favourite soap-opera, the inhabitants of 'Coronation Street' or for the 'Archers'. The old gentleman who is blind but so independent that he wants no help or interference — he's *Water Violet*. And Laura Archer, with all her campaigning is surely a *Vervian* type. Even the Peanuts cartoon characters provide an opportunity for learning about the remedies. Every film or play that has real characterisation can provide a wealth of material. That man whose young son died and he never expressed any grief, just took to heavy drinking — he needed *Agrimony*. The woman who runs the corner shop who won't let you escape before she has told her life story — she's a *Heather* type. What about Eeyore in 'Winnie the Pooh'? He's a classic *Gentian*: remember his comment "Good morning, if it is a good morning which I doubt"?

Shakespeare or Dickens could keep us busy for weeks with theoretical prescriptions. In 'Hamlet' a series of remedies would be called for. The type remedy for Hamlet himself is *Scleranthus* for his indecision ("to be or not to be, that is the question . . ."). Then he would need *Mustard* for his deep melancholia and *Cherry Plum* for his thoughts of suicide and incipient madness. *Aspen* and *Walnut* would have helped him when faced with the ghost of his dead father. Other heroic characters can be analysed in a similar way.

Working like this can be entertaining. A more practical approach entails the observation and analysis of our own psychological states. Think back over your life and it will be easy to see when a particular psychological pattern was prominent. What were you like as a child? Were you irritable and impatient, lacking in confidence, always trying to be cheerful but hiding your worries, overactive, or listless and dreamy? In each case there was a recognisable type remedy indicated. Then remember those periods of crisis and notice the reverberations both psychological and physical. Perhaps there was a time of parting from the familiar home environment, moving house, the loss of a parent, accidents and injuries. Each situation would tell its own story in terms of the remedies that would have been appropriate. Possibly we may be able to recognise the causal pattern between the psychological state and subsequent illness. Perhaps an early love affair went wrong, we were bitterly disappointed and soon afterwards we 'caught' glandular fever. Maybe a leg was broken playing football and afterwards we never had the confidence to play games again and that was the time when we began to get asthma. It may be appropriate to deal with the still latent shock in such a situation by taking *Star of Bethlehem* today. A case that is not untypical involved a man of 30 who still suffered from the trauma of nearly drowning at the age of three.

We may recall other incidents from later life. Was there a time when you were extremely busy and nearly exhausted yourself by over-expending your energy? Conversely there may have been a period when nothing seemed to go right, you felt discouraged and depressed, even to the point where hopelessness took hold. Then we may remember that there was a period of desperation and anguish when everything looked meaningless — in one case such a time of distress led to the loss of all a man's hair, such a condition may still be reversed. We might also see that there were times of great happiness when we were absorbed in a productive and fulfilling occupation, life was delightful and

47

joyous — were we ill then? It is sure that we were not.

Having surveyed our own life in this way and seen which remedies would have been and are still appropriate we will have learned much. Then we could turn our attention to family and friends. No doubt the reader will have already matched a remedy to someone they know. Once we can recognise the quality of one of the type remedies we will see it occur time and again. It is like learning a new word which suddenly seems to be used all the time though we never noticed it before. Recognise one strong characterisation of a type and we always have a sort of cut-out Aunt Sally to check against. Such a characterisation will not have the subtleties of the real thing but it will serve as a reference point. If we can recognise a type remedy in this way then it should be relatively easy to see what transient states are also applicable. Thus a *Vervain* suffering from a *Gentian* condition is quite different to the *Gentian* condition of a *Water Violet*. The *Vervain* may suffer depression energetically with an active outgoing expression (he will kick the cat) while a *Water Violet* will just withdraw more into solitude (you will see even less of him than usual).

So learning to diagnose really entails a study of human nature. It is striking that a person of experience and maturity who is not acquainted with the remedies can nonetheless make an immediate and accurate diagnosis by reference to a textbook. To such a person the descriptions are a formulated expression of what is already known to be so. Those of us who have still much to learn will find that working with the remedies brings a deeper and loving understanding of mankind that can be used in the service of others. For as we are given knowledge so we have a duty to apply ourselves to help our neighbours.

MAKING THE MEDICINE

Having selected the remedies that are needed we must then prepare the medicine. A small clean screwtop bottle, preferably with a dropper (20 or 30 mls is the best size — they can be obtained from a chemist) should be used. Three-quarters fill it with fresh water — it is advisable to use natural spring water though this is not imperative — and then top up with a small teaspoonful of brandy. The brandy acts as a preservative and keeps the remedy clear. It is interesting to note that Bach elected to use brandy since it was related to two of the remedies: it is the fruit of the Vine and is matured in Oak casks. We then take out the stock bottles of the requisite remedies and put two drops of each into the medicine bottle. It is well to take care to keep everything clean so avoid touching the glass of the dropper. Gently shake the medicine bottle to mix the contents and then but for one thing it is ready to be used.

It was Dr Bach's privilege to discover these healing remedies and as we have seen it was an integral part of his outlook upon life that man had to acknowledge his Divine origin and recognise that the greater part of a human being lies beyond the physical body that he inhabits. We are the creation of One God and we should endeavour to live, love and learn in this world as children whose parent is Unity. All healing comes through the Grace of the Almighty and we should petition that the Spirit of Strength and Love may work within the remedy to heal those who are in need of help, so that, if it be Thy Will, we may all live more perfectly to achieve Thy purpose.

So then, let us say a prayer over the remedy before it is passed from our hands. After that, as Edward Bach himself wrote . . .

> There is nothing more to say, for the understanding mind will know all this, and may there be sufficient of those with understanding minds, unhampered by the trend of science, to use these Gifts of God for the relief and blessing of those around them.[3]

BIBLIOGRAPHY

Edward Bach: *The Twelve Healers & Other Remedies.*[3]

——— *Heal Thyself* — An Explanation of the Real Cause & Cure of Disease.

Nora Weeks: *The Medical Discoveries of Edward Bach Physician.*[1]

Philip M. Chancellor: *Handbook of the Bach Flower Remedies.*

Jane Evans: *The Benefits of the Bach Flower Remedies.*

F. J. Wheeler: *The Bach Remedies Repertory.*

T. W. Hyne Jones: *Dictionary of the Bach Flower Remedies.*[2]

All these books are published by The C. W. Daniel Company Ltd.
1 Church Path
Saffron Walden
Essex CB10 1JP
England

Gregory Vlamis: *Flowers to the Rescue.*[4] Thorsons Publishing Group.

Those who wish to obtain further information should write to:

The Dr Edward Bach Centre
Mount Vernon
Sotwell
Nr Wallingford
Oxon OX10 0PZ
England

Lecture tapes and other educational material available from:

Bach Educational Programme
P.O. Box 65
Hereford HR2 0UW